Table of Contents

INTRODUCTION 4

What are the symptoms of a cold? 6

Symptoms   Cold Flu 8

Diagnosing a cold... 9

Treatment for adults 11

Home remedies 13

Treatment for children 14

WHAT FOOD SHOULD YOU EAT IF YOU HAVE A COLD? 16

Risk factors for the common cold.......................... 17

How to protect yourself from a cold 19

How to protect others 20

WHAT CAUSES A STUFFY NOSE? 22

Causes of nasal congestion................................ 23

Home remedies for nasal congestion.............. 24

Treatment for congestion.......................... 26

When you should see a doctor..................... 27

Infants and children................................... 28

HOW TO RELIEVE SINUS PRESSURE............................ 30

OTC remedies 34

10 HOME REMEDIES FOR HELPING TO EASE A RUNNY NOSE ... 37

How to get rid of a runny nose due to an allergy.................. 43

What makes a runny nose go away?............................... 46

How to Clear a Stuffy Nose..................................... 48

Antihistamines or allergy medication........................... 53

WHAT TO KNOW ABOUT SWOLLEN LYMPH NODES
(LYMPHADENOPATHY/ADENOPATHY) 55

What are lymph nodes? 55

Noninfectious causes.. 59

What Does My Type of Cough Mean?................................ 60

Wet cough 63

Dry cough... 66

When to see a doctor 70

CONCLUSION 73

INTRODUCTION

The common cold is a viral infection that affects the upper respiratory tract. The most common cause is a rhinovirus, and the most common symptoms are a stuffy or runny nose, sneezing, and a scratchy, sore throat. The first signs of the common cold are fairly obvious: a stuffy or runny nose, sneezing, and a scratchy, sore throat. Most people quickly recognize these early symptoms because the common cold is so ordinary. In fact, adults have an average of 2 to 3 coldsTrusted Source per year.

The common cold is actually a viral infection in your upper respiratory tract. A cold can be caused by more than 200 virusesTrusted Source. The most common are rhino viruses. These viruses are easily spread from person to person or surface to surface. Many of these viruses can live on surfaces for hours, even days. While the common cold may indeed be familiar, there are some things to know about this ailment that can help you feel better, avoid future colds, or even prevent the spread of the virus to other people.

What are the symptoms of a cold?

Once you're exposed to a cold-causing virus, cold symptoms typically take 1 to 3 daysTrusted Source to appear. The symptoms of a cold rarely appear suddenly. Nasal symptoms include:

congestion

sinus pressure

runny nose

stuffy nose

loss of smell or taste

sneezing

watery nasal secretions

postnasal drip or drainage in the back of your throat

Head symptoms include:

watery eyes

headache

sore throat

cough

swollen lymph nodes

Whole body symptoms include:

fatigue or general tiredness

chills

body aches

low grade fever below 102°F (38.9°C)

chest discomfort

difficulty breathing deeply

Symptoms of a cold typically last for 7 to 10 daysTrusted Source. Symptoms tend to peak around day 5 and gradually improve. However, if your symptoms worsen after a week or haven't disappeared after about 10 days, you may have another condition, and it may be time to see a doctor.

What's the difference between a cold and the flu?

The common cold and the flu may seem very similar at first. They are indeed both respiratory illnesses and can cause similar symptoms. However, different viruses cause these two conditions, and your symptoms will help you differentiate between the two. Knowing the difference between cold and flu symptoms can help you decide how to treat your condition — and whether you need to see a doctor.

Symptoms	Cold	Flu
Symptom onset	gradual (1–3 days)	sudden
Symptom severity	mild to moderate	moderate to severe
Fever	rare	common
Headache	rare	common
Sore throat	common	occasionally
Aches	mild	moderate to severe
Chills	uncommon	common

Cough, chest discomfort	mild	to	moderate
common, can be severe

Sneezing	common	occasionally

Vomiting, upset stomach	rare	occasionally

Complications	rare	occasionally

As a rule, flu symptoms are more severe than cold symptoms.

Another distinct difference between the two is how serious they are. Colds rarely cause additional health conditions or problems. The flu, however, can lead to complications like:

sinus and ear infections

pneumonia

sepsis

Diagnosing a cold

Diagnosing an uncomplicated cold rarely requires a trip to your doctor's office. Recognizing the symptoms of a cold is often all you need in order to figure out your diagnosis. Of course, if your symptoms worsen or last longer than 10 days, make an appointment with a doctor. You could actually be dealing with a different health condition, which your doctor will be able to diagnose. If you have a cold, you can expect the virus to work its way out of your system in about 7 to 10 days.

If your doctor diagnoses a cold, you'll likely only need to treat your symptoms until the virus has had a chance to run its course. These treatments can include using over-the-counter (OTC) cold medications, staying hydrated, and getting plenty of rest. If you have the flu, the virus may take the same amount of time as a cold to fully disappear. But if you notice your symptoms are getting worse after day 5, or if you don't start feeling better after a week, it's a good idea to follow up with your doctor, as you may have developed another condition.

If you have the flu, you may benefit from taking an antiviral flu medication early in the virus' cycle. Rest and hydration are also very beneficial for people with the flu. Much like the common cold, the flu just needs time to work its way through your body.

Treatment for adults

The common cold is a viral infection in your upper respiratory tract. Viruses cannot be treated with antibiotics. In most cases, viruses like the cold just need to run their course. You can treat the symptoms of the infection, but you can't actually treat the infection itself. Cold treatments generally fall into two main categories: over-the-counter (OTC) medications and home remedies.

Over-the-counter (OTC) medications

The most common OTC medications used for colds include:

Decongestants. Decongestant medications help ease nasal congestion and stuffiness.

Antihistamines. Antihistamines help prevent sneezing and also ease runny nose symptoms.

Pain relievers. Nonsteroidal anti-inflammatory drugs (NSAIDs) such as ibuprofen (Advil, Motrin), naproxen (Aleve), and aspirin can help ease body aches, inflammation, and fever symptoms.

Common cold medications sometimes include a combination of these medications. If you're using one, be sure to read the label and understand what you're taking so you don't accidentally take more than you should of any one class of drug. The most common side effects from OTC cold medications include:

dizziness

dehydration

dry mouth

drowsiness

nausea

headache

If you've previously received a diagnosis of high blood pressure, you should consult your doctor before using any OTC cold medications. Certain medications help relieve symptoms by narrowing blood vessels and reducing blood flow. If you have high blood pressure, this may affect blood flow throughout your body.

Home remedies

Like OTC cold remedies, home remedies for the common cold don't cure or treat a cold. Instead, they can help make your symptoms less severe and easier to manage. The most effective and common home remedies for a cold include:

Gargling with salt water. A salt water gargle can help coat your throat and ease irritation.

Drinking plenty of fluids. Staying well hydrated helps you replace fluids you've lost while also helping relieve congestion.

Using vapor rub. Vapor rub topical ointments help open your airways and ease congestion.

Getting lots of rest. Getting plenty of rest helps your body save energy to let the virus run its course.

Zinc lozenges. Zinc lozenges may reduce how long cold symptoms last if they're taken at the very start of your symptoms.

Echinacea. According to research, echinacea may be effective at reducing the duration of a cold in some cases.

Treatment for children

The Food and Drug Administration (FDA)Trusted Source doesn't recommend OTC medications for cough and cold symptoms in children younger than 2 because these medications could cause serious and potentially life threatening side effects. Manufacturers voluntarily label these cough and cold products: "Do not use in children under 4 years of age." You may be able to help ease a child's cold symptoms with these home remedies:

Rest. Children who have a cold may be more tired and irritable than normal. If possible, let them stay home from school and rest until the cold has cleared.

Hydration. It's very important that children with a cold get plenty of fluids. Colds can dehydrate them quickly. Make sure they're drinking regularly. Water is great. Warm drinks like tea can pull double duty as a sore throat soother.

Food. Kids with a cold may not feel as hungry as usual, so look for ways to give them calories and fluids. Smoothies and soups are two good options.

Salt water gargles. Salt water gargles aren't the most pleasant experience, but gargling with warm, salty water can help soothe sore throats. Saline nasal sprays can also help clear nasal congestion.

Warm baths. A warm bath may help ease mild aches and pains that are common with a cold.

A cool mist humidifier. A cool mist humidifier can help decreaseTrusted Source nasal congestion. Don't use a warm mist humidifier, as it can cause swelling in the nasal passages, making it more difficult to breathe.

Bulb syringe. Nasal suctioning with a bulb syringe works well to clear babies' nasal passages. Older children typically resist bulb syringes.

WHAT FOOD SHOULD YOU EAT IF YOU HAVE A COLD?

When you're sick, you might not feel like eating at all, but your body still needs the energy that food provides. The following foods may be extra helpful for your cold recovery:

Chicken noodle soup

The salty soup is a classic "treatment" for all kinds of illnesses. It's especially great for colds. Warm liquids are good for helping open up your sinuses so you can breathe more easily, and the salt from the soup can ease irritated throat tissue.

Hot tea

Warm drinks like tea are great for colds. Add honey for a cough-busting boost. Slices of ginger may also reduce inflammation and ease congestion. Try to stay away from coffee, though. Caffeine can interfere with medications, and it may increase your risk of dehydration.

Yogurt

Yogurt contains billions of healthy bacteria that can boost your gut health. Having a healthy microbiome in your gut may help your body fight any number of illnesses and conditions, including a cold.

Popsicles

Like hot tea, popsicles may help numb and ease the pain of a sore throat. Look for low sugar varieties or make your own "smoothie" pop with yogurt, fruit, and natural juices. The most important thing to remember when you have a cold is to stay hydrated. Drink water or warm tea regularly. Avoid caffeine and alcohol while you're recovering from a cold. Both can make your cold symptoms worse.

Risk factors for the common cold

Certain conditions may increase your risk of catching a cold. These include:

Time of year. Colds can happen any time of year, but they're more common in the fall and winter, or during rainy seasons. We spend more time inside when it's cold and wet, which increases the chance of the virus spreading.

Age. Children under age 6 are more likely to develop colds. Their risk is even higher if they're in day care or a child care setting with other kids.

Environment. If you're around a lot of people, such as on a plane or at a concert, you're more likely to encounter rhinoviruses.

Compromised immune system. If you have a chronic illness or have been sick recently, you may be more likely to pick up a cold virus.

Smoking. People who smoke have an increased risk of catching a cold, and their colds tend to be more severe.

Lack of sleep. Irregular or inadequate sleep can affect your immune system, which may make you more susceptible to cold viruses.

How to protect yourself from a cold

Uncomplicated colds are a minor illness, but they're inconvenient and can certainly make you feel miserable. You can't get a vaccine to prevent colds like you can the flu. But you can do a few key things during cold season to help you avoid picking up a cold virus.

Tips for cold prevention

Wash your hands. Washing your hands with soap and water is the best way to stop the spread of germs. Use alcohol-based hand sanitizer gels and sprays as a last resort when you can't get to a sink.

Avoid sick people. This is reason number one why sick people shouldn't go to work or school. It's very easy to spread germs in tight quarters like offices or classrooms. If you notice someone isn't feeling well, go out of your way to avoid them. Be sure to wash your hands if you come into contact with them.

Take care of your gut. Eat plenty of bacteria-rich foods like yogurt, or take a daily probiotic supplement. Keeping your gut bacteria healthy can help boost your overall health.

Don't touch your face. Cold viruses can live on your body without making you sick, but once you touch your mouth, nose, or eyes with infected hands, you'll likely get sick. Avoid touching your face, or wash your hands before you do so.

How to protect others
When a person contracts a cold-causing virus, it can be spread to others through the air, on surfaces, and through close, personal contact. People carrying the virus can also leave virus behind on shared surfaces like doorknobs and computers. If you're sick with a cold, it's important to be a good neighbor, family member, or friend and take steps to protect those around you when possible.

Tips for protecting others

Wash your hands. Washing your hands protects you, but it also protects others. When you wash your hands, you reduce the risk of spreading the virus elsewhere in your home, school, or workplace.

Stay at home. While you're sick or your child is sick, stay home if possible. You need the rest, and it can help prevent spreading the virus to others.

Avoid contact. Though it may be tempting to show love to another person, it's for their own health that you avoid hugging, kissing, or shaking hands while you're sick. If you must greet someone, try an elbow bump.

Cough into your elbow. If you feel a sneeze or cough coming on, grab a tissue to cover it. If you don't have one, sneeze or cough into your elbow, not your hands. If you accidentally use your hands, wash them immediately.

Disinfect regularly. Pick up a container of disinfecting wipes and give all high touch surfaces, like doorknobs, kitchen counters, appliances, and remotes, a quick cleaning if you or someone in your home is sick.

WHAT CAUSES A STUFFY NOSE?

You may experience nasal congestion due to a viral illness like the flu. But if it lasts longer, it may indicate an underlying health condition, such as allergies or enlarged adenoids. Nasal congestion, also called a stuffy nose, is often a symptom of another health problem such as a sinus infection. It may also be caused by the common cold. Nasal congestion is marked by:

a stuffy or runny nose

sinus pain

mucus buildup

swollen nasal tissue

Home remedies may be enough to alleviate nasal congestion, particularly if it's caused by the common cold. However, if you experience long-term congestion, you may need medical treatment.

Causes of nasal congestion

Congestion is when your nose becomes stuffed up and inflamed. Minor illnesses are the most common causes of nasal congestion. For instance, a cold, the flu, and sinus infections can all cause stuffy noses. Illness-related congestion usually improves within 1-2 weeks. If it lasts longer than 10-14 days, it's often a symptom of an underlying health issue. Some explanations for long-term nasal congestion may be:

allergies

hay fever

noncancerous growths, called nasal polyps, or benign tumors in the nasal passages

sinonasal tumors, though this is rare

chemical exposures

environmental irritants

a long-lasting sinus infection, known as chronic sinusitis

anatomic variants, such as a deviated septum, inferior turbinate hypertrophy, or concha bullosa

enlarged adenoids

gastroesophageal reflux disease, especially in infants

Nasal congestion may also occurTrusted Source during pregnancy, usually during the end of the first trimester. Hormonal fluctuations and increased blood supply that occur during pregnancy may cause this nasal congestion These changes may affect the nasal membranes, causing them to become inflamed, dry, or to bleed.

Home remedies for nasal congestion
Home remedies can help when you're experiencing nasal congestion. Humidifiers that add moisture to the air may help to break up mucus and soothe inflamed nasal passageways. However, if you have asthma, ask a doctor before using a humidifier. Propping your head up on pillows can also encourage mucus to flow out of your nasal passages. Saline sprays are safe for all ages, but for babies you might choose to use an aspirator, or nasal bulb,

afterward, depending on how well the saline flushes out the nasal passages. An aspirator is used to remove any remaining mucus from the baby's nose.

Neti pot

A neti pot is a type of nasal irrigation device that is designed to help flush mucus from the nasal cavity using a saline solution. In addition to a neti pot, nasal irrigation devices are also commonly available as squeeze bottles, which some people may find easier to use.. And These devices are often usedTrusted Source to clear congestion and reduce inflammation, which may be beneficial for those with allergies or an upper respiratory infection. Keep in mind that you should only useTrusted Source filtered or distilled water, as using tap water could increase the risk of infection. Additionally, be sure to clean your neti pot or nasal irrigation device thoroughly after each use, replace it regularly, and talk to a doctor before using the device on children.

Treatment for congestion

After a doctor has determined the cause of chronic nasal congestion, they can recommend a treatment plan. Treatment plans often include over-the-counter or prescription medication to resolve or alleviate symptoms. Medications used to treat nasal congestion include:

oral antihistamines to treatTrusted Source allergies, such as loratadine (Claritin) and cetirizine (Zyrtec)

nasal sprays that contain antihistamines, such as azelastine (Astelin, Astepro)

nasal steroids, including budesonide (Rhinocort), fluticasone (Flonase), or triamcinolone (Nasacort)

antibiotics

over-the-counter or prescription-strength decongestants, including nasal sprays, drops, or tablets

Keep in mind that certain nasal decongestant sprays, such as Afrin, should not be used for more than 3 days in a row, as it could cause nasal congestion to recur or worsen. If you have nasal polyps in your nasal passages or sinuses that are keeping mucus from draining out, a doctor might prescribeTrusted Source oral steroids, allergy medications, steroid rinses, or biologics to help relieve symptoms. In some cases, a doctor may also recommend surgery to remove them.. If there are tumors in your nasal passages, a doctor might perform a biopsy to determine if they are malignant and may recommend surgery for removal. Surgery may also be recommended for a deviated septum if other treatment methods are unable to relieve symptoms.

When you should see a doctor
Sometimes, home remedies aren't enough to relieve congestion, particularly if your symptoms are caused by another health condition. In this case, medical treatment may be needed, especially if your condition is painful and interfering with your everyday activities. If you've experienced any of the following, see a doctor right away:

congestion lasting longer than 2 weeks

congestion accompanied by a high fever lasting more than 3 days

green nasal discharge along with sinus pain and fever

a weakened immune system, asthma, or emphysema

You should also see a doctor right away if you've had a recent head injury and are now having bloody nasal discharge or a constant flow of clear discharge.

Infants and children

Nasal congestion is a common issue in children and infants. However, because infants breatheTrusted Source mostly through their nose during the first few months of life, nasal congestion could potentially interfere with feeding and cause breathing issues, though this is uncommon. For these reasons, it's best to contact a pediatrician right away if your infant has nasal congestion. This is especially important for infants under 3 months old and those with other symptoms, such as a persistent cough, fever, or breathing problems.I will The pediatrician can then work with you to find the best treatment options for your baby.

Outlook

Nasal congestion rarely causes major health problems and is most often caused by the common cold or a sinus infection. Symptoms usually improve right away with proper treatment. If you experience chronic congestion, speak to a doctor to investigate the underlying problem and determine the best course of treatment.

HOW TO RELIEVE SINUS PRESSURE

You can relieve sinus pressure with the help of natural remedies like a humidifier, saline washes, and biofeedback. But you may need medical attention if your symptoms do not improve after a week or two. Sinus pressure results from blocked nasal passages. When your sinuses cannot drain, you may experience inflammation and pain in your head, nose, and face. Many people experience sinus pressure from seasonal allergies or the common cold. While some over-the-counter (OTC) treatments can help reduce symptoms, there are also many effective natural remedies.

1. Steam

Dry air and dry sinuses can increase sinus pressure, causing sinus headaches and pain. Steam can add moisture to the air, moisten your sinus passages, and thin out mucus that may have thickened over time. Some ways to breathe in moistened air include:

taking a hot shower

breathing over a cup of tea

using a humidifier

2. Eucalyptus

If your sinus pressure is related to a viral infection, you can try adding eucalyptus oil to your bath or vaporizer to help speed your recovery. Eucalyptus contains cineole, an ingredient that mayTrusted Source speed the healing of viral sinusitis. The oil also may help to reduce nasal stuffiness and clear your pathways.

3. Saline flush

You can do a sinus flush at home to relieve sinus pressure and congestion. A sinus flush uses sterile saltwater rinsed through your nasal passages to wash away debris and allergens. You can also try saline nasal spray contains salt that helps to increase moisture in your nose and reduce sinus pressure. You can buy sterile saline spray in drugstores or make your own with baking soda, distilled water, and iodine-free salt. If making your own, you must use distilled water, filtered water, or water that has been boiled, as other sources may contain harmful bacteria.

4. Rest

A good night's sleep can help the body to heal. Also, when you're at rest, your body can produce more white blood cells, which help you recover from viruses and other bacteria. Allowing your body to rest can help to reduce sinus pressure, speed your recovery time, and leave you feeling more refreshed. If your sinus pressure makes sleeping difficult, check out these tips for sleeping with a cold that may help.

5. Elevation

Just as sleep is essential for healing, how you sleep can improve or worsen sinus symptoms. Lying flat can increase mucus buildup in your nasal passages, increase your sinus pressure, and disrupt your sleep cycle. Prop your head with pillows at night to keep your head above your heart. This sleeping position can help prevent sinus buildup and allow you to breathe more comfortably.

6. Hydration

Dehydration can contribute to your sinus passages drying out and increased pressure on your face. Increase your water intake throughout the day if you feel under the weather. Fluids will reduce blockages in your sinuses. While water may be your first choice to remain hydrated, you can also retain fluids through other foods and beverages, including:

broth/ soups

ice cubes

herbal tea

water-based vegetables and fruits, like cucumber and watermelon

7. Relaxation

Your sinus pressure may cause you to feel tension in your head, face, and neck. Relaxation may help relieve some headaches. You can try incorporating deep breathing exercises and meditation to achieve relaxation and reduce pain. Yoga, meditation, and other relaxation techniques can help to reduce pain and pressure from sinus infections.

8. Exercise

Similar to yoga, exercise can reduce sinus pressure. Physical activity can increase blood circulation and temporarily relieve congestion to ease breathing. Although uncomfortable to perform while sick, low impact physical activity can help to improve your recovery time and speed healing. This can include taking a walk or doing gentle yoga.

9. Warm compress

You can place a warm compress, such as a washcloth dampened with warm water, over your sinuses to relieve swelling. This may help open your nasal passages.

OTC remedies

If home remedies do not work, you may also be able to relieve sinus pressure with common OTC products. These can depend on the cause of your sinus pressure and may include:

nasal decongestants, such as pseudoephedrine

antihistamines, if allergies are causing your sinus pressure

vapor rub, which can make you feel as though you are breathing better

expectorants, which can break up mucus

Outlook

Sinus pressure symptoms can be painful and uncomfortable. In addition to using traditional treatment methods like decongestants and pain relievers, alternative home remedies can also boost your recovery. If you continue to experience sinus pressure symptoms after two weeks, or if they begin to worsen, seek medical attention. This could indicate a more severe infection that may require prescribed antibiotics.

Home Remedies for a Runny Nose

Home remedies that help you stay hydrated and keep the nasal area moist can make you feel more comfortable if you have a runny nose. Treatment can also depend on the underlying cause. A runny nose is caused by excess mucus production in your nasal passages. This leads to watery secretions that drip from your nose and sometimes also drip down the back of your throat. A runny nose can occur with or without nasal congestion, also known as a stuffy nose. Nasal congestion is caused by inflammation of the lining of your nasal passages, which makes it harder to breathe through your nose.

There are a few reasons why you might have a runny nose. The most common is a viral infection of the sinuses — typically the common cold. In other cases, a runny nose may be due to cold weather, allergies, sinusitis, or other causes. When you breathe in a virus or an allergen like dust or pollen, it irritates the lining of your nasal passages and sinuses. This causes your nose to start making clear mucus that traps the germs or allergens and helps flush these harmful substances out of your nose.

10 HOME REMEDIES FOR HELPING TO EASE A RUNNY NOSE

On its own, a runny nose isn't usually a cause for concern. If you don't have any other symptoms, there are several ways to manage a runny nose at home with natural self-care options that don't involve medication. Let's take a closer look at some of the at-home treatments that may help a runny nose.

1. Drink plenty of fluids

Drinking fluids and staying hydrated when dealing with a runny nose can be helpful if you also have symptoms of nasal congestion. This ensures that mucus in your sinuses thins out to a runny consistency and is easy for you to expel. Otherwise, it may be thick and sticky, which can make your nose more congested. Avoid beverages that dehydrate rather than hydrate. This includes drinks like coffee and beverages containing alcohol.

2. Hot teas

On the other hand, hot beverages like tea may sometimes be more helpful than cold ones. This is because of their heat and steam, which help open and decongest airways. Certain herbal teas contain herbs that are mild decongestants. Look for teas that contain anti-inflammatory and antihistamine herbs, such as chamomile, ginger, mint, or nettle. Make a cup of hot herbal tea (preferably noncaffeinated) and inhale the steam before drinking. Sore throats often accompany runny noses — drinking hot herbal tea can help soothe a sore throat, too.

3. Humidifier

According to a 2019 study, inhaling warm steam from a humidifier significantly improves mucus buildup caused by allergic rhinitis. Similarly, a 2015 study of people with the common cold found that using steam inhalation was quite effective. It reduced illness recovery time by about 1 week compared to no steam inhalation at all. Humidifiers work by transforming water into vapor to moisten otherwise dry air. When you breathe in moisture, it helps to thin and dislodge mucus and soothe irritated sinuses. If you decide to use a humidifier, it's important to clean it regularly according to the manufacturer's instructions. Otherwise, it can become a breeding ground for microorganisms such as mold and bacteria, which can exacerbate sinus problems.

4. Facial steam

Much like a humidifier or a hot cup of tea, a facial steam can help loosen mucus and relieve your runny nose. Here's how to do it:

Heat water in a clean pot on your stove, just enough so that steam is created — DON'T let it reach a boil.

Place your face about 8 to 12 inches above the steam for about 5 minutes at a time. Don't let your face touch the water. Close your eyes and take deep breaths through your nose. Take breaks if your face gets too hot.

Blow your nose afterward to get rid of mucus.

Repeat the process 2 or 3 times a day if you still have symptoms.

If desired, add a few drops of decongestant essential oils to your facial steam water. About 2 drops per ounce of water is sufficient.

Eucalyptus, peppermint, pine, rosemary, sage, spearmint, tea tree (melaleuca), and thyme essential oils are great options. Compounds in these plants (like menthol and thymol) are also found in many over-the-counter (OTC) decongestant. If you don't have these essential oils, you can use these herbs in dried form instead. Make your facial steam into an herbal tea and inhale the vapors — you'll get the same benefits.

While research suggests there are health benefits, the FDA doesn't monitor or regulate the purity or quality of essential oils. It's important to talk with a healthcare professional before you begin using essential oils and be sure to research the quality of a brand's products. Always do a patch test before trying a new essential oil.

5. Hot shower

Need some quick relief? Try a hot shower. Just like humidifiers and facial steam, a shower's hot vapors can help alleviate a runny and stuffy nose. Place your face and sinuses directly in the steam and spray of the shower for best results.

6. Neti pot

Using a neti pot for nasal irrigation (also called nasal lavage) is a common approach to sinus issues. This includes runny nose problems and discomfort. Neti pots are small teapot-like containers with a spout. You add a warm saline or saltwater solution to the pot and then pour the solution through one nostril and out the other. This rinses out your sinuses quite thoroughly. You can purchase a neti pot kit at your local pharmacy, store, or online. Make sure to follow directions for your neti pot exactly. Improper use of neti pots can, on rare occasions, make runny noses worseTrusted Source or cause sinus infections. Make sure to use sterile and distilled water rather than tap water.

7. Nasal spray

Nasal sprays are a common OTC treatment for a runny nose. While medicated nasal sprays are available, saline nasal sprays are a natural treatment to help rinse the nose. Much like nasal irrigation, they target nasal congestion and mucus using gentle salt water. According to a 2021 study of people with upper respiratory infections, the use of a saline nasal spray improved symptoms including a runny nose, nasal congestion, and sleep quality. You can purchase a saline nasal spray at a neighborhood pharmacy or online.

8. Warm compress

Applying a warm compress or washcloth to your forehead and nose several times per day may help improve your runny nose and soothe sinus pressure. A warm compress works by boosting blood circulation in your sinus area. A washcloth or wet compress can help break up nasal stuffiness by adding moisture to the air you breathe. To make your own warm compress at home, soak a clean cloth in hot (not boiling) tap water and place it across your forehead and nose for 15 to 20 minutes. Reapply as needed.

9. Eating spicy foods

Spicy foods can make a runny nose worse. However, if you're also having symptoms of nasal congestion, eating spicy foods may help. If you can tolerate a bit of heat in your food, give it a try. If you're unaccustomed to spiciness, try a small amount of spicy seasoning at first to see if it helps. Hot spices like cayenne pepper, ghost pepper, habanero, wasabi, horseradish, or ginger are great options. These spices, while also creating a feeling of heat when eaten, dilate passageways in the body and can relieve sinus issues.

10. Capsaicin

Capsaicin is the chemical that makes chili peppers spicy. It's been used to treat nerve pain and psoriasis, but if you apply it on your nose, it can help with a runny nose caused by congestion. Several studies have found that capsaicin is more effective at treating runny noses than the OTC medication budesonide.

How to get rid of a runny nose due to an allergy

When a runny nose is caused by an allergy, the easiest way to clear it up is to avoid the allergen. For example, if you are allergic to ragweed, stay inside on days when ragweed pollen counts are high. Instead of opening your windows, use a fan or air conditioner to cool your home. Keep in mind, however, that it's not always possible to completely avoid allergens. If you're allergic to pet dander, for instance, you might not be able to avoid all contact with pets. Still, limiting contact or removing yourself from the situation will typically relieve your symptoms. Other common allergy treatments to clear up a runny nose caused by an allergy include the following OTC and prescription drugs:

antihistamines

nasal and/or oral corticosteroids

nasal sprays

If you have a severe allergy, your doctor might suggest other treatments, such as allergy drops.

Tips for coping with a runny nose

A runny nose is a sign of an immune system reaction. Your immune system is working, which could leave you feeling more tired than usual. Although you might not have other symptoms, you should still go easy on yourself. To cope with a runny nose, try the following:

Get lots of rest. Make sure your runny nose doesn't get in the way of your sleep — take a shower before bed or use a humidifier in your bedroom.

Stay hydrated. To prevent dehydration, make sure you're taking in plenty of fluids.

Blow your nose. Use a soft tissue to wipe or blow excess mucus from your nasal passages. Moisturize the skin around your nose to help prevent soreness.

Wash your hands. Avoid spreading germs by frequently washing your hands with soap and water.

Disinfect surfaces. Take a moment to wipe down surfaces and items that you touch regularly with a disinfectant.

Stay home. Even if you don't have other symptoms, it's a good idea to stay home when you have a runny nose so you don't get others sick.

Frequently asked questions

How do I stop a runny nose fast?

The only way to stop a runny nose fast is to blow your nose, as this will temporarily remove mucus from the nasal passage. Applying capsaicin may help clear the nasal passages for a while. If your runny nose is due to an allergy, antihistamine tablets may help.

What makes a runny nose go away?

The only way to make a runny nose go away is by treating the underlying cause, such as an allergy. If it is due to a cold or flu, you will have to wait until the infection runs its course.

How long do runny noses last?

This will depend on the cause. If it stems from an allergy, the symptoms should improve when you move away from the allergen. A cold usually clears up in 7–10 daysTrusted Source. If symptoms last more than 10 daysTrusted Source, you may have sinusitis, an inflammation of the sinuses. In this case, it may be a good idea to see a doctor.

Why is my nose running like water?

A runny nose that is very watery may be due to an allergy, eating spicy food, or being out in cold weather. Viral and bacterial infections are more likely to produce thicker mucus.

There are many home remedies you can try to get relief from a runny nose without using medication. None of these remedies are designed to actually cure or completely get rid of the underlying cause of a runny nose — namely colds, viral infections, or allergies.These approaches will only give you relief. Make sure to seek more direct treatment if you're experiencing colds, viruses, and allergies, or have other concerning symptoms.

How to Clear a Stuffy Nose

A stuffy nose can be due to mucus or inflamed blood vessels in your sinuses and often develops when you're sick. Other than taking medications, several home remedies can help unclog your nose. A stuffy nose, or nasal congestion, can be frustrating and often affect your day-to-day life. Many people think a stuffy nose results from too much mucus in the nasal passages. However, a clogged nose is usually the result of inflamed blood vessels in the sinuses. A cold, the flu, allergies, or a sinus infection can all inflame these blood vessels. Regardless of the reason for your stuffed-up nose, there are easy ways to relieve it.

Use a humidifier

A humidifier can be a quick and easy way to reduce sinus pain and help relieve nasal congestion. The machine converts water to moisture that slowly fills the air, increasing the humidity in a room. Breathing in this moist air can soothe irritated tissues and swollen blood vessels in your nose and sinuses. Some people claim that heated, humidified air can also help congested mucus drain better.

However, reviewsTrusted Source have shown that there's no current evidence to support this. If you're experiencing symptoms of nasal congestion, you may still benefit from placing humidifiers around your house or office.

Take a shower

Have you ever had a stuffy nose and found that you could breathe so much better after a hot shower? There may be a good reason for that. Steam from a shower may helpTrusted Source to thin out the mucus in your nose and reduce inflammation. Taking a hot shower can help your breathing return to normal, at least for a little while. You can get the same effect by breathing in steam from hot water in a sink. Here's how:

Turn on the hot water in your bathroom sink.

Once the temperature is right, place a towel over your head and put your head over the sink.

Allow the steam to build, and take in deep breaths.

Be careful not to burn your face on the hot water or steam.

Learn more about steam inhalation for congestion relief here.

Stay hydrated

It's important to drink plenty of fluidsTrusted Source if you suspect you have a cold or are experiencing flu symptoms. Maintaining optimum hydration levels can help thin the mucus in your nasal passages, pushing the fluids out of your nose and decreasing the pressure in your sinuses. Less pressure means less inflammation and irritation. If you're also experiencing a sore throat, warm liquids like tea may be able to help ease the discomfort in your throat, too.

Use a saline spray

Take hydration one step further with saline, a saltwater solution. Using a nasal saline spray can increase the moisture in your nostrils. Some saline sprays also include decongestant medication. Talk with your doctor before you begin using saline sprays with decongestants.

Drain your sinuses

It's not glamorous, but you can clean out your clogged nostrils with a Neti pot. A neti pot is a container designed to flush mucus and fluids out of your nasal passages. The Food and Drug Administration (FDA)Tmrecommends using distilled or sterile water instead of tap water. Here's how to use a neti pot:

Stand with your head over a sink.

Place the spout of the neti pot in one nostril.

Tilt the neti pot until water enters your nasal passage.

Once the water flows into your nostril, it will come out through your other nostril and empty into the sink.

Do this for about 1 minute, and then switch sides.

Learn more about the correct ways to use a neti pot to relieve congestion here.

Use a warm compress

A warm compress may help alleviate some symptoms of nasal congestion by opening the nasal passages from the outside. To make a warm compress, first, soak a towel in warm water. Next, squeeze the water out of the towel, then fold it and place it over your nose and forehead. The warmth can provide comfort from any pain and help relieve the inflammation in the nostrils. Repeat this as often as necessary.

Take medications

A congested nose can be uncomfortable, but some other over-the-counter (OTC) medications may clear out your nasal passages and bring relief. Make sure to speak with a pharmacist when choosing a decongestant, antihistamine, or allergy medication. The pharmacist can also answer any questions you may have about a particular medication.Call your doctor if your stuffy nose doesn't improve after taking medication for more than 3 days, or if you have a fever as well.

Decongestants

A decongestant medication can help reduce swelling and ease pain associated with irritated nasal passages. Many decongestants are available without a doctor's prescription. They come in two forms: nasal spray and pill. Common decongestant nasal sprays include oxymetazoline (Afrin) and phenylephrine (Sinex). Common decongestant pills include pseudoephedrine (Sudafed, Sudogest). Be cautious when using decongestants. You shouldn't take a decongestant for more than 3 days without a doctor's supervision. After 3 days, a nasal decongestant may actually make your congestion and stuffiness worse. In addition, people with high blood pressure (hypertension) should not take typical decongestants. Safe alternatives are available, but it may be best to speak with your doctor to assess which medication is right for you.

Antihistamines or allergy medication

You may want to take an antihistamine or allergy medication if your nasal congestion results from an allergic reaction. Both types of medications can reduce the swelling in your nasal passages, helping to unclog your sinuses. Combining drugs containing both an antihistamine and a decongestant can relieve the sinus pressure and swelling caused by allergic reactions. Follow the instructions for these medications carefully. If you don't, you may make your condition worse. You should also note that antihistamines might make you drowsy. If you aren't sure how an antihistamine will affect you, don't take this medication when you need to be active or productive.

Nasal congestion, which many people refer to as a stuffy nose, is the result of inflammation of blood vessels in your sinuses. If you are experiencing symptoms of nasal congestion, there are a number of home remedies you can try. These include hot showers, warm compresses, and various OTC medications.

WHAT TO KNOW ABOUT SWOLLEN LYMPH NODES (LYMPHADENOPATHY/ADENOPATHY)

Lymph nodes are small glands that filter lymph, the clear fluid that circulates through the lymphatic system. During an infection, they accumulate bacteria or dead or diseased cells and may swell. When a person has an infection, they may notice swollen lymph nodes in part of the body near the infection site, such as their neck, armpit, jaw, or groin. For instance, a person with a sore throat due to COVID-19 may have swollen lymph nodes in their neck. They may also have other symptoms of an infection, such as coughing, fatigue, and fever. Cancer that develops in or spreads to the lymph nodes may also be swollen. In this case, the reason for swelling may be a tumor.

What are lymph nodes?

The lymphatic system consists of channels throughout your body that are similar to blood vessels. Lymph nodes are small glands that filter lymph, the clear fluid that circulates through the lymphatic system. Lymph nodes are located throughout the body. They can be found underneath the skin in many areas, including:

in the armpits

under the jaw

above the collarbone

on either side of the neck

on either side of the groin

Lymph nodes store white blood cells, which are responsible for killing invading organisms. They also act like a checkpoint. When bacteria, viruses, and abnormal or diseased cells pass through the lymph channels, the lymph nodes detect and stop them. When faced with an infection or illness, the lymph nodes accumulate debris, such as bacteria and dead or diseased cells.

How do you know if you have swollen lymph nodes?

Lymphadenopathy is another name for swelling in the lymph nodes. Symptoms that may be present along with swollen lymph nodes in the neck, for instance, are:

coughing

fatigue

fever

chills

runny nose

sweating

Swollen lymph nodes in the groin may occur with a pelvic infection. They can cause pain when walking or bending.

What does a swollen lymph node indicate?

Swollen lymph nodes are one sign that your lymphatic system is working to rid your body of infection and illness.

Infections

Lymph nodes swell when an infection occurs in the area where they're located. For example, the lymph nodes in the neck can become swollen in response to an upper respiratory infection, such as the common cold. Lymph nodes that swell due to an infection may beTrusted Source painful. Swollen lymph nodes in the head and neck may stem from infections such as:

ear infection

sinus infection

the flu

strep throat

mononucleosis (mono)

tooth infection, including an abscessed tooth

skin infection

HIV

Sexually transmitted infections (STIs) such as syphilis or gonorrhea can bring about lymph node swelling in the groin area. Other possible causes include:

cat scratch fever

tonsillitis

toxoplasmosis

tuberculosis

shingles

Noninfectious causes
Serious conditions, such as immune system disorders or cancers, can cause lymph nodes throughout the body to swell. Immune system disorders that cause the lymph nodes to swell include lupus and rheumatoid arthritis. Any cancers that spread in the body can cause the lymph nodes to swell. When cancer from one area spreads to the lymph nodes, the survival rate decreases. Lymphoma, which is a cancer of the lymphatic system, also causes the lymph nodes to swell. Cancers that can cause swollen lymph nodes include:

leukemia

Hodgkin's lymphoma

non-Hodgkin's lymphoma

Sézary syndrome, a rare type of lymphoma

Other causes of swollen lymph nodes include, but aren't limited to:

some medications, such as antiseizure and antimalarial drugs

allergic reactions to medications

stress

gingivitis

mouth sores

What Does My Type of Cough Mean?

Coughing can involve an involuntary reflex that kicks in when your body attempts to remove irritants, or coughing can be done voluntarily. It can be a symptom of illness or due to an obstruction in the airway. Coughing usually occurs because of an irritation in your throat or airway. When this occurs, the nervous system sends a message to your brainstem. Your brainstem responds by telling the muscles in your chest and abdomen to contract and expel a burst of air, producing a cough. A cough protects your body from irritants such as:

mucus

smoke

allergens, such as dust, mold, and pollen

Keep reading to learn about different types of coughs and the illnesses or conditions that may cause them.

Classifying types of coughs

Coughing is a common symptom of many types of medical conditions and illnesses. You may be able to determine the cause of your cough by its characteristics. Coughs can be described by:

Behavior or experience: When and why does the cough happen? Does it occur at night, after meals, or during exercise?

Characteristics: How does your cough sound or feel? Hacking, wet, or dry?

Duration: How long have you had your cough? Has it been less than 2 weeks or more than 8 weeks?

Associated effects: Do you have other symptoms such as vomiting, urinary incontinence, or sleeplessness?

Grade: How bad is it? Is it annoying, persistent, or debilitating?

Sometimes, an obstruction in your airway may trigger your cough reflex. If you or your child has swallowed something that may be blocking the airway, seek immediate medical attention.

Choking

If you notice any of these signs in your child, call 911 or your local emergency services immediately and perform the Heimlich maneuver or begin CPR. Signs of choking can include:

bluish skin

loss of consciousness

inability to speak or cry

wheezing, whistling, or other odd breathing noises

weak or ineffective cough

panic

Note that the maneuver for babies (less than 12 months old) who are choking is different. Learn how to help a choking baby.

Wet cough
A wet cough is also referred to as a productive cough because it commonly involves bringing up mucus from the lungs. The If you are experiencing a wet cough, it may feel like there's an object in the back of your throat. It may also feel like something is dripping into your throat or chest. Some of your coughs may bring mucus up into your mouth. The following conditions can cause a wet cough:

common cold or the flu

pneumonia

chronic obstructive pulmonary disease (COPD), chronic bronchitis, or emphysema

acute bronchitis

asthma

The duration of your cough may be a big clue as to its cause. Wet coughs can be acute, lasting for fewer than 3 weeksTrusted Source, or chronic, lasting more than 8 weeksTrusted Source in an adult.

Wet coughs are often accompanied by other symptoms such as:

runny nose

postnasal drip, or the excess mucus that drips from your nose into your throat

fatigue

Wet coughs sound wet because of the moisture present when mucus comes up from your respiratory system. In situations where babies, toddlers, and children have wet coughs, the coughs are nearly always caused by either a cold or the flu.

Remedies for a wet cough

Adults: Adults can use over-the-counter (OTC) cough and cold medications for acute wet coughs, and some people may use honey to ease cough symptoms.

Babies and toddlers: A cool mist humidifier can help relieve dryness in the surrounding air. It may also be helpful to use saline drops in your child's nasal passages and then use a bulb syringe to clean the nose. Do not give any type of OTC cough or cold medication to babies or toddlers under age 2. It's also not safe to give honey to children under age 1Trusted Source due to the risk of infant botulism.

Children: A clinical trialTrusted Source found that giving 1 1/2 teaspoons of honey a half-hour before bedtime can reduce cough and improve sleep in children ages 1 and older. You can also use a humidifier during the night to keep the air moist. You should speak with your doctor first if you want to use any OTC cough and cold medications as a treatment.

If your cough persists for more than 3 weeks, you may need to talk with a doctor about other treatments. A child's wet cough is considered chronic after 4 weeksTrusted Source.

A dry cough is a cough that doesn't cause any mucus to come up. It may feel like you have a tickle in your throat. This can trigger your cough reflex and cause hacking coughs. Dry coughs can be challenging to manage, and they may turn into long coughing fits. Dry coughs typically occur when there is inflammation or irritation in the respiratory tract, but there isn't very much or any mucus to cough up. Dry coughs can be caused by upper respiratory infections, including a cold or the flu.

Dry cough

Dry coughs may linger for several weeks or until a cold or the flu has run its course. Other potential causes of dry cough can include:

laryngitis

sore throat

croup

tonsillitis

sinusitis

asthma

allergies

gastroesophageal reflux disease (GERD)

medications, especially ACE inhibitors

exposure to irritants such as air pollution, dust, or smoke

COVID-19 and dry cough

A dry cough is a common symptom of COVID-19.

If you're sick and think you may have COVID-19, the Centers for Disease Control and Prevention (CDC)Trusted Source recommend the following:

Stay home and avoid public places.

Isolate from your family members and pets as much as possible.

Cover your coughs and sneezes.

Wear a mask if you have to be around other people.

Stay in touch with a doctor.

Call ahead if you end up seeking medical attention.

Wash your hands often.

Avoid sharing any personal or household items with other people.

Disinfect common surfaces often.

Monitor your symptoms.

When it's an emergency

If you experience any of the following symptoms, seek emergency medical attention:

trouble breathing

heaviness or tightness in the chest

bluish lips

confusion

Was this helpful?

Remedies for a dry cough

Remedies for dry cough can depend on its cause.

Adults: If you have a dry cough, throat lozenges, cough suppressants, staying hydrated, or using a humidifier may provide some relief.

Babies and toddlers: In babies and toddlers, dry coughs don't usually require treatment. A humidifier may help make them feel more comfortable. For relief from croup, you can bring your child into a bathroom full of steam or outside in the cool night air.

Older children: You can use a humidifier to help prevent their respiratory system from becoming too dry. Older children may be able to use cough drops to soothe their sore throats.

If you have symptoms such as heartburn or pain in addition to a dry cough, you should speak with a doctor. You may need a prescription for antibiotics, asthma medications, or antacids, or you may need further testing to determine the cause of your cough. If you are taking any supplements or medications, make sure that you tell the doctor about them.

If a child's cough continues for longer than 2–3 weeks, speak with your doctor to determine possible causes. Your child may need a prescription for antibiotics, asthma medications, or antihistamines.

When to see a doctor

Often, coughs do not require a doctor's visit. Whether you need to see a doctor depends on what type of cough you have and how long you have had it, as well as your age and health.

Those who are living with certain lung diseases, such as asthma and COPD, may need earlier or more frequent treatment. Children who are experiencing a cough should see a pediatrician or another healthcare professional if they:

have a cough that continues for more than 3 weeks

have a prolonged or high feverTrusted Source

become so out of breath that they can't talk or walk

turn bluish or pale

are dehydrated or unable to swallow food

are extremely fatigued

make a "whoop" sound while coughing violently

are wheezing in addition to coughing

When it's an emergency

Call 911 or your local emergency services if your child:

loses consciousness

cannot be awakened

is too weak to stand

Adults who are experiencing a cough should see their doctor if they:

have a cough that lasts for more than 3–8 weeks

cough up blood

have a fever above 100.4°F (38°C)

are too weak to talk or walk

are severely dehydrated

make a "whoop" sound while coughing violently

are wheezing in addition to coughing

have daily acid reflux or a cough that interferes with sleep

When it's an emergency

Call 911 or your local emergency services if an adult:

loses consciousness

cannot be awakened

is too weak to stand

There are many types of coughs. The specific characteristics, severity, and duration of a cough may help pinpoint the cause. Coughing is a symptom of many illnesses and can be caused by a variety of conditions.

CONCLUSION

The average common cold lasts anywhere from 7 to 10 daysTrusted Source, but they can last as long as 2 weeksTrusted Source. Depending on your overall health, you may have symptoms for more or less time. For example, people who smoke or have asthma may experience symptoms for a longer period of time. If your symptoms don't ease or disappear within 7 to 10 days, make an appointment to see a doctor. If your symptoms begin worsening after 5 days, it's also important to see a doctor. Symptoms that don't go away or get worse could be a sign of a bigger problem, such as the flu or strep throat.